# BEFORE YOU GO UNDER

# BEFORE YOU GO UNDER

## A step by step guide to ease your mind before going under anesthesia

### BENJAMIN TAIMOORAZY, M.D

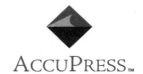

ACCUPRESS™

Published by Accupress LLC in Association with Before You Go Under™

First Printing: February 2008

Printed in the United States of America

P.O. Box 5095 Bloomington IL 61702

Phone: (309) 660-2976      Fax: (309) 661-8132

To order please visit www.beforeyougounder.com

    An Accupress Edition

ACCUPRESS™

ISBN 978-0-615-18470-8

Library of Congress Control Number: 2008900310

WARNING & DISCLAIMER

This book is intended to provide general information regarding a reader' s fears and concerns regarding anesthesia. It is not intended as a substitute for the reader', s own research and investigation. This book is not intended to replace the advice of reader' s medical physician regarding any prior or anticipated medical procedure. This book is not intended to be a substitute for medical information or diagnosis concerning reader' s current medical condition. The author and publisher shall have neither liability nor responsibility to any person or entity with respect to any loss or damage caused or alleged to be caused directly or indirectly by information contained in this book. The author and publisher have checked with sources believed to be reliable and accurate at the time of publication. However, in view of the possibility of human error and/or changes in medical science, neither the author nor publisher warrants that the information contained herein is in every respect accurate or complete. The reader is encouraged to confirm the information contained herein with other sources. The names of organizations, products or procedures appearing in this book are given for information purposes only.

Cover Design and page layout by Edmond Oushana, AccuPress LLC.

*Dedicated to all my patients who were the driving force for this endeavour, to the unknown heroes of the operating room as their efforts make miracles possible, to my parents who crossed the oceans in pursuit of a better future for their children,*

*and*

*especially to my wife, Ramica
and my daughters, Tiffany and Nicole
for making it all worthwhile.*

# Acknowledgements

I would like to extend my deepest Appreciation and gratitude to *John Moody* for editing this manuscript so enthusiastically, and to *Deborah Peters*, *MadeLon Gay Dolan,* and *Linda Leinhart* for their constructive input and support for this project.

In particular I wholeheartedly wish to thank *Edmond Oushana* for his dedicated work in preparing all the graphic design materials and the countless hours he spent in putting it all together. This book could not have been produced without their hard work and dedication.

# Contents

*"Nothing has such power to broaden the mind as the ability to investigate systematically and truly all that comes under thy observation in life."*

**Marcus Aurelius**

# INTRODUCTION

Every year in the United States more than 30,000,000 surgical procedures are performed under anesthesia. This means that every six to seven years, one of us may need to be rolled into that cold, unfamiliar chamber filled with high-tech gizmos and instruments called the operating room. There we entrust our lives, handing over full authority and control to highly trained professionals, albeit for a short period of time. In some instances, life-saving decisions are made in seconds and that is when all those decades of training and experience come into play.

For most of us, it is that feeling of losing control and the fear of the unknown that make this experience a rather freaky one. But wait. Like everything else, when you shed light on the problem, you will start to understand it, analyze it, and in the case of anesthesia and surgery, you may even start to appreciate what the science of medicine has achieved to provide us with a smooth sailing through what historically has been one of the most challenging obstacles in human physiology.

In my 14 years of practice as an anesthesiologist, I have come across people from all walks of life and backgrounds. From superstitious to highly educated, analytic personalities, from easy going to the worry wart. We all have concerns when faced with surgery. Some of us deal with our fears and concerns quietly, and the rest of us express ourselves more openly, seeking answers and reassurances.

***"I don't want to feel anything or hear anything when I am in surgery. What***

*if I don't wake up? I hate needles. I am claustrophobic. I get really sick after anesthesia. I may be pregnant. I have allergies. How do you know that I am adequately anesthetized?"*

These are but a few of the questions and comments made by most of us as we face the seemingly unknown world of anesthesia. And one can only appreciate the ever escalating levels of concern as the air waves and television screens are flooded with anesthetic related horror stories. Through the years, as I see patients prepare to undergo a surgical procedure, amazingly many of the same concerns are echoed.

Therefore, I felt compelled to work on a manuscript that would address, in simple terms, the most commonly asked questions and alleviate concerns by explaining some of the misconceptions related to the anesthetic experience. This information should also provide you with the peace of mind that going under anesthesia is safer than ever. *"BEFORE*

*YOU GO UNDER"* is the result of this effort. The information provided in this manuscript will not only shed light on the events that occur behind the closed doors of the operating room, but also will empower you with the knowledge to ask all the pertinent questions, assuring delivery of quality health care that you deserve. Having said that, let us begin to relieve your anxieties, clear the air of the mist of misconceptions, and let science be your guide to excellent surgical and anesthetic outcomes.

*"There is a single light of science, and to brighten it anywhere is to brighten it everywhere."*

**Isaac Asimov**

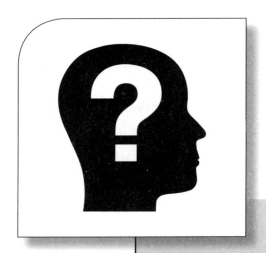

*What is anesthesia?*

# What is anesthesia?

## 1

The word "anesthesia" (from the Greek language) means loss of sensation. In 1846, Oliver Wendell Holmes best defined anesthesia as "a sleep-like state that makes possible painless surgery." Discovery of anesthesia is a totally American contribution to the science of medicine. Anesthesia is basically a temporary loss of feeling or awareness induced by medications allowing surgery to be performed painlessly. This may be provided by blocking the sensation to a small part of the body, to total unconsciousness or general anesthesia. Depending on the type of surgery and your general medical history, your anesthesiologist can help you decide which type of anesthesia is best suited for you.

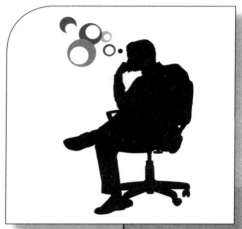

*What are the different types of anesthesia?*

# What are the different types of anesthesia?

Depending on the type of your surgical procedure and your general medical condition, your anesthesiologist can help you decide which type of anesthesia is best suited for you. The following describes different types of anesthesia you may elect for your surgery.

## General Anesthesia

General anesthesia is a complete loss of consciousness induced by a combination of injected and or inhaled drugs. Under general anesthesia you have no pain and no memory of the operative events. Your anesthesia provider will monitor the progress of surgery and by adjusting the dosage of anesthetic medications assures that adequate depth of anesthesia is maintained. To provide you with general anesthesia, once you are in the pre-surgical area, an intra-

10

venous line is started; this will allow your anesthesiologist to provide you with a dose of a relaxant medication to take your mind off the events. From there, you are wheeled into the operating room (usually on a gurney) and monitors for blood pressure, electrocardiogram and breathing are placed on you. Before the anesthetic medications are administered, your anesthesiologist will ask you to breathe some oxygen, usually using a face mask. Some patients with claustrophobia may find this experience rather uncomfortable. So, if you suffer from this condition, make sure to ask to be sedated with intravenous medications before the application of the face mask. The next thing you know, you are waking up in the recovery room. There you will be monitored for approximately one hour after surgery for adequacy of pain control, stability of your vital signs and lack of nausea and vomiting.

## Local anesthesia

Local anesthesia is usually used to perform minor procedures such as stitching, skin biopsies, dental procedures, and breast biopsies. Using a very tiny needle, local anesthesia is accomplished by injecting medications (usually local anesthetics) into the targeted surgical site, resulting in a localized temporary numbness lasting between one to four hours.

## Conscious sedation

This type of anesthesia is used for procedures such as colonoscopy and other endoscopy procedures, cataract removal or placement of a cardiac pacemaker. During the procedure, intravenous sedatives are used. You remain conscious but fully relaxed, with no perception of pain and usually with no recollection of the surgical events.

## Regional anesthesia

The most commonly used regional anesthetic techniques are SPINAL and EPIDURAL anesthetics. They produce numbness, usually from the waist down, and are used for lower abdominal surgeries, urinary bladder operations, Caesarian sections, hips, and lower extremity surgeries. You may elect to stay conscious but will be free of pain. Intravenous medications can be used in conjunction with regional anesthesia to keep you relaxed and sleepy during the procedure.

## Epidural anesthesia

Epidural anesthesia is achieved when local anesthetics are injected into the epidural space which covers the spinal cord and the nerve roots. In most cases, after some intravenous sedation, a tiny plastic catheter is placed in your lower back.

This can be used to deliver local anesthetics into the epidural space, providing you with pain relief for the surgery. The epidural catheter can be kept for up to five days and is an excellent pain control approach for major abdominal and chest surgeries. It is important to point out that the epidural catheter is so tiny that its presence in your back will not restrict your activities in any shape or form.

## Spinal anesthesia

The fear of paralysis after spinal anesthesia is a thing of the past as spinal anesthesia is performed at the lower lumbar levels where the spinal cord has already ended and only nerve roots are present.

Spinal anesthesia is performed either in the sitting position or when you are placed on your side. Some intravenous sedatives are given to you usually prior to the procedure. Once local anesthetics are injected, the results are almost immediate: numbness from your waist down and profound temporary (one to four hours) weakness in your legs. Keep in mind that you will be kept relaxed and sleepy for the duration of the surgery, and all of your vital signs will be continuously monitored by your anesthesia provider. At the conclusion of the operation you will be observed for about one hour in the recovery room to assure the stability of your vital signs. This area is immediately adjacent to the oprtating room and is designated to take care of you after surgery. The average length of stay in the recovery room is about one hour.

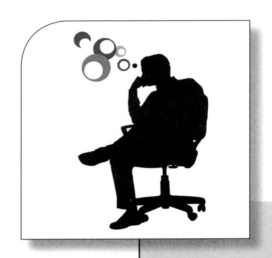

*How does anesthesia work?*

# How does anesthesia work?

## 3

Anesthesia is a temporary interruption of nerve function. General anesthesia works by selective reversible depression of brain function, resulting in a sleeplike state, with freedom from pain and presence of profound amnesia. The new medications used for induction and maintenance of general anesthesia have a shorter stay in the body systems; therefore, once their administration is ended you wake up faster and with much less grogginess. By the same token, local anesthesia works by temporary interruption of nerve function at the injection site. So, if injected near peripheral nerves (in your arm or in your leg), they cause numbness in that extremity. And, if injected into the spine, it results in spinal or epidural anesthesia, making you feel numb from waist down. The duration of action of local anesthetics depends on the type of medication used and can range between one to four hours.

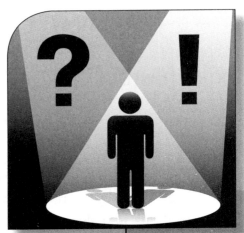

*How do you know that I am adequately anesthetized?*

# How do you know that I am adequately anesthetized?

## 4

This is one of the most frequently asked questions and a source of a great deal of anxiety and concern among patients undergoing surgical procedures. This topic also has been one of the most intensely studied and debated subjects in the field of anesthesiology. As discussed in chapter one, anesthesia is a temporary loss of feeling or awareness induced by medications allowing surgery to be performed painlessly. This may be provided by blocking the sensation to a small part of the body, to total unconsciousness or general anesthesia. Depending on the type of the surgical procedure and your general medical condition, different anesthetizing choices are available.

If surgery is being performed under local anesthesia, adequacy of anesthesia is evaluated by ensuring the targeted surgical site is completely numb after injecting anesthetic medication. In the case of spinal or epidural anesthesia, the adequacy of anesthesia is verified by the absence of perception of pin-prick sensation when a rather pointed object is applied to your skin at the surgical site.

The ultimate judge of adequacy of anesthesia in both of these circumstances is the patient who will acknowledge the presence of numbness after anesthesia is provided. In most cases, at this point, intravenous sedative medications are administered to keep the patient relaxed and sleepy while undergoing surgery. But one cannot argue the fact that once under general anesthesia, verification of adequacy and depth of anesthesia are the sole responsibilities of the anesthesiologist.

During general anesthesia, brain function and memory formation are the targets of anesthetic medications, providing you with a sleeplike state devoid of pain or the memory of the surgical procedure. To monitor the adequacy of depth of anesthesia, your anesthesiologist is equipped with a profound knowledge of human physiology and a variety of monitoring devices that directly or indirectly measure the depth and impact of anesthesia on your body and brain function.

To achieve adequate depth of general anesthesia, your body weight, age and presence of co-existing medical conditions are used to calculate the type, dosage and concentration of anesthetic medication. At the same time, the impact of these medications is monitored by fluctuations of your blood pressure, heart rate and breathing pattern, and necessary adjustments are made continuously throughout the course of the operation.

In recent years, with the introduction of a brain wave monitoring device, the science of anesthesiology and our capability to objectively monitor the depth of general anesthesia has taken a major leap forward. Once general anesthesia is administered (either by intravenous medications or by inhaling the anesthetic agent), the impact of the medications and the depth of anesthesia are monitored by connecting you to this device using a sticky pad placed on your forehead. The numeric readout on this monitor reflects the depth of anesthesia: the smaller the number the deeper the anesthetic.

In summary, it is only by combining the information retrieved from all of the aforementioned monitoring devices and from the fluctuations of your vital signs (blood pressure, heart rate, etc.) that your anesthesiologist will have the capability to determine the depth of anesthesia with a high degree of accuracy, providing you with peace of mind and comfort during your surgical procedure.

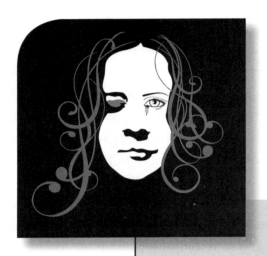

*Awareness under anesthesia*

# Awareness under anesthesia

## 5

Awareness under anesthesia is a rare but devastating complication associated with general anesthesia. Every now and then this complication becomes a matter of front page news, as the air waves, movie and TV screens suddenly are flooded with horror stories of patients who were awake during surgery. But the fact is, awareness under anesthesia is a well recognized and intensely studied entity in the field of anesthesiology. And for every surgical procedure, your anesthesiologist makes plans well in advance to prevent this feared companion of surgery and anesthesia.

To better understand the etiology of awareness under anesthesia, it is prudent to explain the sequence of events and steps taken to induce, maintain and terminate the general anesthesia process. As explained in chapter two, general anesthesia is a complete loss of consciousness induced by a combination of injected and or inhaled drugs. Some of these medications will put you to sleep and the others, like muscle relaxants, will provide adequate exposure for the surgeon in the operative field. It takes a few seconds for these medications to exert their anesthetic effects as they have to reach the brain (the target organ for anesthesia). Once under general anesthesia, you should have no pain and no memory of the operative events. Anesthetics in general have depressant effects on cardiovascular and respiratory systems. So as anesthesia is induced there is a predictable drop in blood pressure, rate of breathing and heart rate. In a patient with normal or near normal cardiovascular and pulmonary function, these changes are well tolerated. In some instances however, your anesthesiologist has to provide the necessary support to maintain your vital signs by interventions such as placing a breathing tube (to support respiration) and administration of intravenous medications (to support circulation). Other factors such as chronic consumption of alcohol and pain killers, sedatives and other forms of drug abuse can dramatically alter the dosage requirement of the anesthetics.

Having said that, the following describes the most common conditions associated with awareness under anesthesia:

1-Usage of muscle relaxants(paralytic medications) during surgery: In the presence of muscle relaxants, the patient is unable to move or react to the pain of surgical incision if adequate anesthesia is not provided.

2-Acute emergencies such as fetal distress during pregnancy: When salvaging of the fetus is so urgent that there is not enough time to establish adequate depths of anesthesia.

3-Severely compromised cardiovascular conditions: For example after motor vehicle accidents or acute heart attack, when the blood pressure is so low that body cannot tolerate additional depressant effects of anesthetics on the cardiovascular system.

To monitor the depth of anesthesia, a variety of direct and indirect indices are used. These include: Fluctuations of your blood pressure, heart rate, breathing patterns and eye movement. The levels of the anesthetic medications are also monitored in your exhaled gases. However, the most significant breakthrough in the science of monitoring depth of anesthesia is the introduction of the brain wave monitoring device. This monitor provides the only objective means of measuring the impact of anesthesia on the brain. The device is connected to the patient by placing a sticky monitoring pad on the forehead, and a numeric readout reflects the depth of anesthesia. The smaller the number, the deeper is the level of anesthesia.

Whatever the cause, awareness under anesthesia is a devastating experience and every effort should be made to support the patient psychologically and emotionally and to determine the reasons for its occurrence. Together with other monitoring devices, the brain wave activity monitor is an intricate and priceless component of the weapons available to combat the problem of awareness under anesthesia. It is a good idea to ask your anesthesiologist if the surgical facility is equipped with this device. There is nothing to lose and much to gain in implementing every available tool to safeguard your surgical experience against the dangers of awareness under anesthesia.

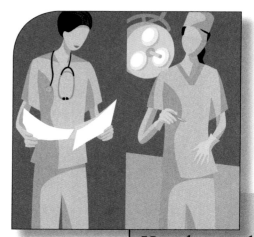

*How does one become an anesthesiologist or a nurse anesthetist?*

# How does one become an anesthesiologist or a nurse anesthetist? 6

Anesthesiologists are physicians, who after graduating from medical school or school of osteopathy, enroll in an intensive, four year residency training in the specialty of anesthesiology. Anesthesiologists may also become sub specialized in obstetrics, pediatrics, cardiovascular, critical care, chronic pain management or neurosurgical anesthesiology. Today, the scope of practice of anesthesiology has expanded well beyond working in the operating room. It ranges from caring for critically ill patients in the intensive care unit to managing chronic and debiliting painful conditions such as cancer pain and chronic low back pain.

In some facilities anesthesiologists may work as a team with Certified Registered Nurse Anesthetists (CRNAs). To become a CRNA, the candidate must earn an RN or registered nurse degree, work one year as a critical care or recovery room nurse and then complete two years of anesthesia training in an approved nurse anesthesia training program. In some medical centers, CRNAs work under the supervision of the anesthesiologist, and in other institutions, they may work independently.

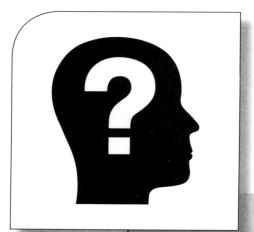

*What is the risk of a major anesthetic complication during my surgery?*

# What is the risk of a major anesthetic complication during my surgery? 7

In the last 25 years, due to the introduction of new anesthetic medications and improved monitoring devices, the risk of anesthetic related complications and mortality has been drastically reduced. Keep in mind that the risk of death from motor vehicle accidents is 45 times higher than that of anesthesia deliveries. As previously mentioned, anesthesia is a temporary and reversible interruption of nerve and mental activity; as soon as its administration is terminated the effects of the anesthetic will rapidly wear off.

However, it should be pointed out that co-existing medical conditions such as severe heart or lung problems, kidney disease, high blood pressure, history of stroke, and carotid artery occlusion can increase the risk of anesthetic related complications. For that reason, if you suffer from any of these conditions, your anesthesiologist will want to see you in advance of your scheduled surgical procedure. He or she will make sure that coexisting medical conditions are evaluated and proper medical management is undertaken. You can also increase the safety of the anesthetic by losing weight, cessation of smoking, and abstaining from alcohol intake.

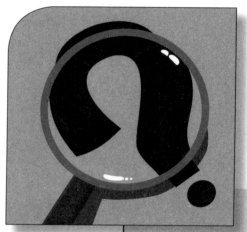

*Do I need anesthesia
for this procedure?*

# Do I need anesthesia for this procedure?

# 8

This is a great question. The answer is that some procedures can be performed safely without anesthesia. For example, even in a claustrophobic patient, with proper preparation, (wash cloth over the eyes, a headset playing your favorite music, and taking a relaxant pill), the MRI procedure can be performed without the need for anesthesia. However, the majority of surgical procedures need to be performed under some form of anesthesia.

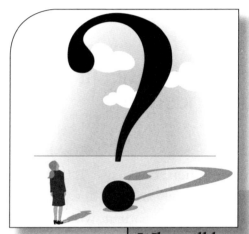

*Who will be my
anesthesia provider?*

# Who will be my anesthesia provider?

## 9

Most of the time you may need to go for your preoperative evaluation days in advance of your scheduled surgery. The anesthesiologist on duty will pay a visit and will ask you questions regarding your medical history and will explain the anesthetic procedure. This does not mean that he or she will be the one to provide you with the anesthetic on the day of your surgery. But don't worry, everything will be well documented from this visit, and on the day of surgery, the anesthesiologist in charge will pay another visit and will review all the information with you one more time. During this visit, he or she will answer any last minute questions you may have and makes sure everything is in perfect order for the best outcome for your operation.

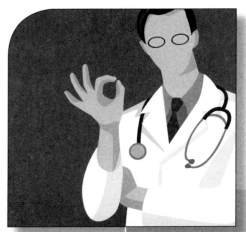

*The responsibility for explanation of the surgical procedure*

# The responsibility for explanation of the surgical procedure

## 10

Once you are seen in your surgeon's office and the decision is made for a specific procedure, it is the surgeon's responsibility to clearly explain the risks and benefits of the procedure, as well as the possibility of potential complications, and answer all the questions you may have. Every surgeon's office must provide you with written materials specific to each procedure, which are usually very informative. It is a good idea to write down your questions and concerns so that you do not feel "lost in the moment" during your visit. Do not hesitate to call back if you have any doubts or questions.

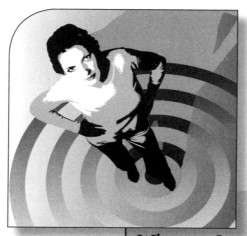

*When am I supposed
to show up for my surgery?*

# When am I supposed to show up for my surgery?

## 11

Your surgeon's office should provide you with the specifics of when and where to appear for your surgery. Normally, you need to be present about 90 minutes in advance if your surgery is in a hospital setting and 30-40 minutes early if it is in an outpatient surgery center. But, of course, if before your surgery more tests or a work up is needed, the surgeon's office will notify you of your arrival time at the healthcare facility.

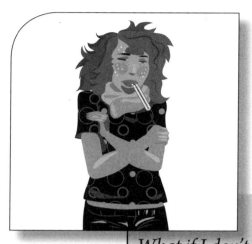

*What if I don't feel well before my surgery?*

# What if I don't feel well before my surgery?

## 12

Your surgeon's office provides you with a list of instructions in preparation for your procedure. If your basic state of well being has changed prior to your surgery, you should immediately inform your health care provider of this change. In some instances such as acute onset of chest pain, severe headache or unusual bleeding, you should contact emergency medical services. In other instances, if you feel like you are coming down with a cold, or you are running a fever, it is wise to inform your health care provider of such change. In these instances it may be necessary to postpone the surgery, since these could be signs of an acute infection.

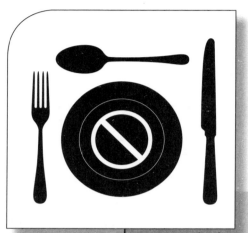

*Fasting before elective surgery*

# Fasting before elective surgery

## 13

The significance of fasting is that when you undergo anesthesia and subsequent surgical procedure on an empty stomach, there is less incidence of nausea and vomiting after surgery and less risk of inhaling stomach contents (liquid or soid) when you are anesthetized. The recommendations for minimum fasting period before anesthesia are as follows:

1-Clear liquids (black coffee, tea, water, soda, and pulp free juices), 2 hours

2-Infant formula, 6 hours

3-Breast milk, 4 hours

4-Solid food, 6 hours

You are allowed to take your morning medications, as directed by your physicians with a few sips of water, 2 to 3 hours prior to your procedure.

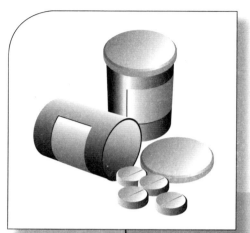

*When should I take my daily medications if I am scheduled for surgery?*

# When should I take my daily medications if I am scheduled for surgery?

## 14

This is a very open-ended question, since the list and diversity of medications is so vast. A good rule of thumb is to take your pills with a few sips of water, 2-3 hours prior to the scheduled surgery. You should ask your health care provider specifically when and which medications to take before your surgery, as taking some may be mandatory while others should be put on hold.

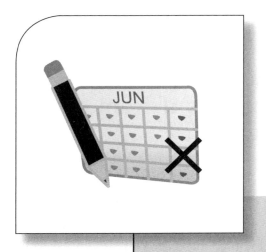

*Surgery cancellation*

# Surgery cancellation

=========================================== **15**

For most patients, surgery cancellations are a very disappointing experience, as patients go through tremendous psychological (the anticipation of getting over the illness), financial (scheduling time off from work), and emotional preparation before surgery. Surgery cancellation is equally bothersome to your doctors and the health care facility, as they also have deadlines to meet, and they arrange their work schedule around you. Sometimes there is a tremendous negative financial impact on the healthcare facility due to surgery cancellation. Common reasons for cancellation of a procedure include the following:

1-You were not fasting long enough before your surgery

2-Your blood work, electrocardiogram, or chest X-ray revealed an unanticipated abnormality

3-Your general medical condition suddenly has changed. Such as sudden experience of chest pain or shortness of breath

4-Failure to arrive on time for the procedure

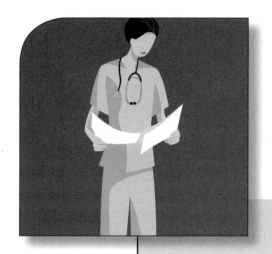

*Medical history*

# Medical history

**16**

Providing an accurate and up to date medical history to your anesthesiologist is paramount for smooth sailing through your surgery and anesthetic experience. Co-existing medical conditions and the medications used in their treatment can have a tremendous impact on anesthetic and surgical outcomes.

Make sure to point out the history of previous surgeries, any adverse reactions during previous anesthetic procedures, allergies and a current list of your medications with their dosages. Having the list of your medications written on a piece of paper is a good practice. Be sure to include all prescription and non prescription medications, including those which you only take intermittently, for example pain killers. It is very crucial to point out the usage of any over the counter supplements. Many over the counter herbal supplements interact significantly with anesthetics and need to be discontinued two to three weeks prior to your planned anesthesia and surgery.

You need also to cover any co-existing medical conditions with your surgeon and anesthesiologist, so they can tailor the procedure and medications accordingly.

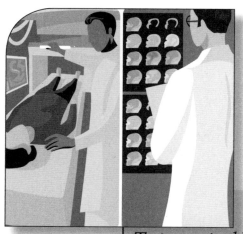

*Tests required before
your planned surgery*

# Tests required before
# your planned surgery

This depends on the type of surgery, your age, and presence
of any underlying medical conditions. The spectrum may
range from no tests required if you are healthy and scheduled to undergo a minor procedure, to a comprehensive
gamut of testing, such as, electrocardiogram (EKG), chest
X-ray, blood work, cardiac work up, such as stress test, and
Computerized Tomography (CT-scan) or Magnetic Resonance Imaging(MRI scanning). The results of the tests will
be reviewed in advance of the planned procedure, and necessary interventions will be implemented. This among other
things may include, adding , removing or adjusting dosages
of your medications, or may even necessitate further testing and work-up to clearly demonstrate how your body will
perform under anesthesia.

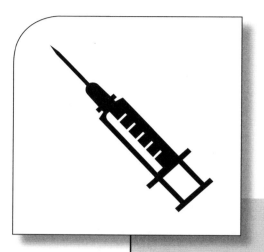

*I hate needles*

# I hate needles

Don't worry. You are not alone. For most people, fear of starting the intravenous line far exceeds anything else that may happen during surgery. This problem may be more complicated in patients with tiny veins, and in small kids when fat can make finding veins even more difficult.
Here are a few helpful hints that will make this experience more pleasant.

1-Ask the health care provider to numb the vein before starting your intravenous line. This can be done by providing you with an anesthetic cream that you need to apply per instruction to specific targeted sites a few hours prior to starting the IV. Alternatively, medical personnel may use a local anesthetic spray applied to the IV site to numb the skin.

2-Keep your arms and hands warm as it will dilate the veins

and makes them easier to find.

3-Drink enough fluids as allowed per instructions to keep fully hydrated.

4-Lie down as they are starting your IV. Always look away and use some kind of distraction to take Your mind off the experience.

5-Recently the use of a device called the vein finder has revolutionized the process of getting an itravenous access. This is based on either ultrasound or near infra-red beam technologies. The latter works by shinning a video image of the patient's vein on top of the skin and takes the guess work out of the picture.

6-Transillumination: This technology is also employed to facilitate pin pointing hard to find veins. It utilizes ultra bright beam of light that penetrates the skin and visualizes hard to find veins on all skin types.

7-And last but not least, you always have the option to request your anesthesia provider to help facilitate this process.

So if starting your intravenous line has historically been

difficult, following these recommendations may make this process a breeze. Being able to find and hit the right vein the first time can make all the difference in the world.

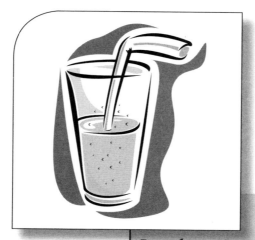

*I am fasting according to the instructions, but I am really thirsty*

# I am fasting according to the instructions, but I am really thirsty

## 19

This is a very common complaint, but unfortunately you are not allowed to drink any kind of fluids within two hours of your surgery and anesthetic. But as soon as your intravenous line is started, an adequate amount of fluid will be given to you to make up for the time you have been unable to drink. Unfortunately, this will not treat the psychological aspect of the thirst sensation and feeling of dry mouth. The good thing is that you don't have to put up with this discomfort for long, as your wait time to undergo your surgical procedure is usually rather brief.

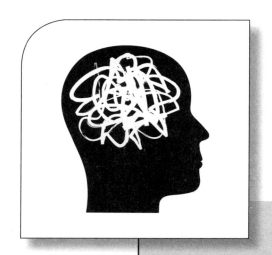

*Anxiety relief before anesthesia*

# Anxiety relief before anesthesia

## 20

It is normal to feel anxious and sometimes really apprehensive about the whole experience of surgery and anesthesia. For some of us it is the feeling of losing control and the fear of unknown outcomes that is really scary.

But ease your mind. Just ask your friendly anesthesiologist to write an order for an anxiolytic (medications that relieve anxiety) as soon as you show up for your procedure. If you still feel anxious, you can have an extra dose of that medication. Remember, this is your show and you are the "superstar" for a day. So, make sure to get the best out of it.

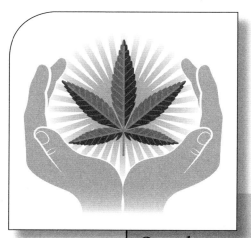

*Over the counter
herbal supplements*

# Over the counter herbal supplements

## 21

Many adults use a variety of herbal supplements, and believe it or not, the majority fail to inform their health care provider of this fact. Some of the most commonly used herbal supplements are: Ephedra, Ginkgo, Ginger, Kava Kava, St.John's Wort, Ginseng, Saw palmetto and Valerian.

Herbal medications and supplements can interact adversely with anesthetics. They may increase the risk of bleeding, produce electrolyte imbalances, cause changes in your blood pressure and circulation and may even keep you sleepy longer than expected after your anesthetic. Therefore, please inform your health care provider of what herbal supplements you are taking. Typically, it is recommended to discontinue their usage at least 2-3 weeks prior to your scheduled anesthetic.

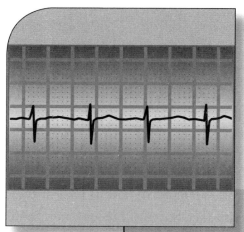

*Monitoring of your vital Signs during surgery and anesthesia*

# Monitoring of your vital signs during surgery and anesthesia

## 22

There are specific recommendations regarding the monitoring of vital signs to be followed during any anesthetic procedure. It is required that qualified anesthesia personnel shall be present in the operating room throughout the conduct of the anesthetic. Also during all anesthetics, your oxygen levels (by using a device called the pulse oxy meter that fits on your finger), your breathing, and your circulation (with monitoring your EKG and blood pressure), shall be continuously monitored. The introduction of cerebral brain wave monitoring has revolutionized the science of evaluating the depth of anesthesia. This device provides the anesthesiologist with a numeric readout, describing the varying levels of consciousness. The smaller the number, the deeper is the levels of anesthesia. The implementation and advances in monitoring of the vital signs is the main reason behind the increase in safety of anesthesia and better outcomes after surgical procedures.

*Why is the operating
room always cold?*

# Why is the operating room always cold?

## 23

Interestingly, this is the most commonly asked question by patients the moment they are rolled into the operating room. To reduce the risk of proliferation of germs, operating rooms are equipped with special air ducts to circulate the air in a specific direction. The temperature is kept on the cool side because the operating room staff must wear special sterile gowns, masks and caps to prevent infection. This is complicated by working under the intense and warm beam of operating room lights, which are used to provide enough visibility for the surgical procedure. A drop in body temperature during surgery is closely associated with increased risk of bleeding, slow awakening from anesthesia and higher than normal incidence of infection in surgical patients. Therefore, maintaining normal body temperature is of paramount importance to your anesthesiologist. This is usually achieved by using electric warming blankets and intravenous fluid warmers.

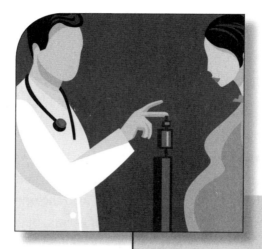

*Pregnancy and anesthesia*

# Pregnancy and anesthesia

## 24

Every year in the United States more than 50,000 pregnant patients undergo non delivery related surgical procedures.

It is imperative to inform your health care provider if you think you might be pregnant. Elective surgery should be avoided at all costs during pregnancy, since both anesthesia and surgical procedures are associated with a higher incidence of preterm labor. During the first trimester there is an especially higher risk of affecting the development of the fetus. Every effort should be made to postpone elective surgical procedures for pregnant patients, unless the risk of postponement puts the mother and fetus at risk. If surgery cannot be avoided, a regional anesthetic technique (depending on the type of the procedure), such as spinal or epidural, is probably the best choice as they least affect the fetus. During pregnancy, narcotics are probably safe medications to be considered for controlling pain after surgery.

Keep in mind that there is always the possibility that you may undergo anesthesia in the early stages of pregnancy. Therefore, many institutions recommend routine pregnancy testing for females of child-bearing age before elective surgery.

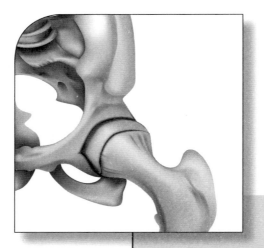

*Artificial implants and surgery*

# Artificial implants and surgery

## 25

Be sure to inform your health care provider if you have any kind of artificial implants. These could be among other things, artificial cardiac pacemakers, artificial joints, and artificial heart valves. The presence of any foreign body, as described above, puts you at a higher risk for infection at the site of the implant and you may need a special antibiotic treatment before your surgery.

It is crucial to know the material used in the making of the implant since performing an MRI procedure is contraindicated in the presence of some of these implants. It is generally safe to do an MRI if the implants are made of titanium. However, presence of artificial cardiac pacemakers, pain management pumps and wires and cochlear implants, is a contraindication to performing an MRI.

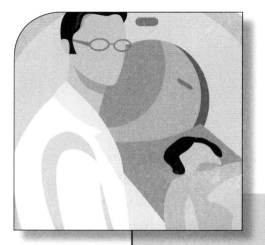

*Claustrophobia*

# Claustrophobia

## 26

Claustrophobia is a rather common condition. This is an anxiety disorder that involves a fear of enclosed or confined spaces. Many develop the condition as a result of being trapped in uncomfortable situations such as a stalled elevator or an overcrowded room, with no easy route to escape.

In some patients with claustrophobia, placing the face mask before starting anesthesia may be uncomfortable. Ask your anesthesia provider to keep you well sedated in advance of this experience.

Having to undergo an MRI procedure is probably the most daunting experience for a claustrophobic patient. But don't worry, you are not alone. Interestingly, many patients experience moderate to severe anxiety during an MRI procedure.

There are many things we can do to alleviate this situation. If you are about to undergo MRI testing, inform your health care provider that you suffer from claustrophobia. In most cases an anesthesiologist is consulted who will explain the procedure and discuss available options for helping you relax during the procedure. Simple interventions may help you undergo your MRI test comfortably and smoothly. These include placing a washcloth over the eyes or using headsets to listen to your favorite music during the procedure.

Additionally, ask if the medical center owns an open MRI machine, which eliminates the sensation of being in a confined space for the most part. Always remember, even in the conventional MRI machine, you are in a confined space but it is not enclosed by any means. Finally, you will have the option to undergo the procedure under twilight conditions. Your anesthesiologist can use very short acting medications to keep you sedated so that you will not see or remember the MRI procedure as it is being performed.

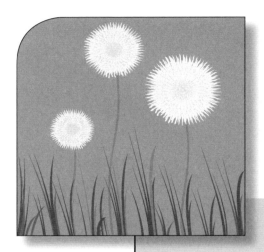

*Allergies*

# Allergies

## 27

Providing your medical team with any information regarding medication or food allergies is quite important. Never assume anything. What you may consider a benign or only a minor problem may lead to serious or even a life threatening reaction during your surgery. It is important to know that some of the medications used for providing anesthesia may cause an allergic reaction, especially when you have food allergies (such as bananas, peanuts, eggs, avocados). Allergic reactions can be prevented by avoiding certain medications or by pre treatment with antihistamines and steroids.

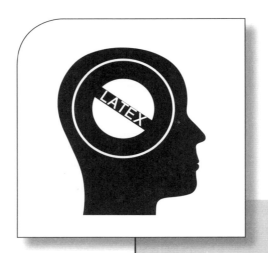

*Latex allergy*

# Latex allergy

## 28

Latex comes from a liquid in tropical rubber trees. It is processed to make different rubber products such as balloons, surgical gloves, pacifiers, rubber bands, condoms, and adhesive tapes. The protein in the rubber can cause an allergic reaction in some people. Latex allergy is a rather common condition especially in healthcare providers. Constant exposure to common household items such as rubber gloves and rubber toys could precede this condition. The spectrum of reactions to latex can range from life threatening allergic reaction (Anaphylaxis) to contact reactions such as itching, rash or hives. If you have other allergies such as hay fever and are constantly exposed to latex, your chances of developing latex allergy are increased. Because some proteins in rubber are similar to food proteins, some foods may cause an allergic reaction in people who are allergic to latex. The most common of these foods are: banana, avocado, chestnut, kiwi fruit, and tomato.

To determine if you have an allergy to latex, a skin test can be performed, but it carries some risk of severe allergic reaction during testing. Therefore, usually performing a blood test to determine the presence of antibodies to latex is preferred.

Always remind your health care provider if you are allergic to latex, as nowadays every medical facility should be equipped with latex free equipments and supplies. If you are allergic to latex, it may be reasonable to provide you with a course of antihistamines and steroids to reduce the severity of a reaction. If you have a history of anaphylactic reaction to latex, you may need to wear a medical alert bracelet.

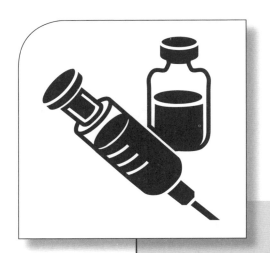

*Antibiotics before surgery*

# Antibiotics before surgery

## 29

Prevention of infection is of utmost importance after a surgical procedure. Even when performed while observing strict sterile techniques, any surgery carries a risk of infection. It is imperative to inform your health care provider of allergies and the type of reactions you might have to specific antibiotics, as alternative choices are available. Usually antibiotics need to be started immediately before the actual surgical incision is made. If you have implants such as artificial cardiac pacemakers or cardiac defibrillators, prosthetic joint replacements, screws or rods in your bones or artificial heart valves, then antibiotics before surgery are not only necessary for preventing infection in the wound, but they will also prevent infection at the site of the implant.

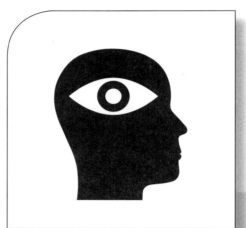

*I don't want to feel anything
or hear anything when
I am under anesthesia*

# I don't want to feel anything or hear anything when I am under anesthesia  30

Well that is a very reasonable request. But keep in mind that some procedures such as cataract surgery, colonoscopy, breast biopsies, and numerous other procedures are performed under sedation and not general anesthesia. So, while fully relaxed, sedated and free of pain, you may hear some of the conversations in the operating room. That is why your anesthesia provider will adjust the medications to provide you with the utmost comfort and amnesia for the procedure. But, when you are under general anesthesia, it is a completely different ball game.

From the concentration and dosage of the medications used, to fluctuations of vital signs, your anesthesiologist can gauge the adequacy and the depth of the anesthetic. Additionally a device, which monitors brain activity, can provide valuable information on how deeply you are anesthetized.

Some physicians believe that the advent of this device has

revolutionized the ability to gauge the level of consciousness, as this is the only monitoring equipment that provides a numerical readout, directly reflecting the depth of the anesthetic.

Keep in mind, that there is not one device or method that can with 100% accuracy reflect the depth of the anesthetic. It is the clinical judgment of your anesthesiologist, combined with the usage of data retrieved from all of the monitoring devices that can provide the necessary information regarding the depth of the anesthetic and smooth sailing through your surgical and anesthetic experience.

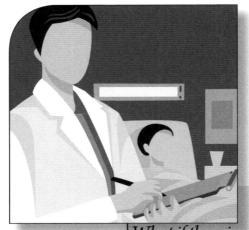

*What if there is a*
*Do Not Resuscitate*
*(DNR) order in my file?*

# What if there is a Do Not Resuscitate (DNR) order in my file?

# 31

Medically and ethically, it is profoundly important to respect the patient's wishes as defined in the advanced directives and the power of attorney for health care.

As previously explained, anesthesia is a temporary interruption and alteration of mental function, and its impact is either reversible or spontaneously resolves upon termination of administration of the anesthetic. But complications do occur as rare and infrequent as they may be. Therefore, advanced directives gain paramount importance as patients with DNR status have to undergo procedures requiring the administration of anesthetics.

In these instances, a special consent form must be signed by the patient or the power of attorney for health care. This defines the level of intervention to resuscitate in case of a complication during your operation.

So, please discuss this very critical medical/legal fact well in advance of your planned surgical and anesthetic procedure, so that proper documentation is reflected in your medical file.

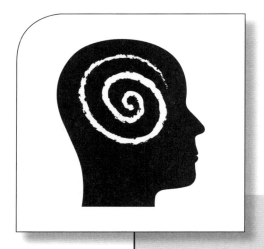

*Motion sickness*

# Motion sickness

## 32

This condition is closely related to nausea and vomiting after anesthesia. Motion sickness is due to oversensitivity of the inner ear to bodily movements which then sends signals to the nausea center of the brain. This may be the most common cause of nausea and vomiting during the ride home after your surgery. Be sure to inform your anesthesiologist about this condition, as specific medications can prevent this abnormality, complicating your recovery from anesthesia and surgery.

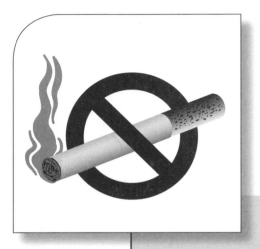

*Smoking and anesthesia*

# Smoking and anesthesia

## 33

Smoking basically increases the risk of cardiopulmonary complications after anesthesia. Smoking increases carbon monoxide levels in the bloodstream which causes difficulty providing oxygen to the heart, brain, and other vital organs of the body. Chest infections are more common in smokers, which may cause uncontrolled coughing spells, resulting in rupture of a surgical wound. It may also delay wound healing and increase the risk of infection at the surgical site, prolonging the recovery after surgery. Interestingly there is an increased dosage requirement for anesthetic medications in smokers.

It is surprising to know that only 48-72 hours of abstinence from smoking can reduce the incidence of pulmonary problems after surgery. But for the best results, you need to quit smoking 8-12 weeks prior to your anesthetic.

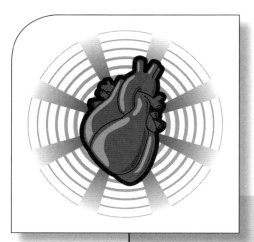

*Anesthesia and*
*co-existing diseases*

# Anesthesia and co-existing diseases

# 34

Generally it is considered safe to proceed with your planned anesthesia and surgery once your underlying medical condition is well under control. Those with co-existing medical conditions may carry a higher risk of anesthetic or surgical complications than other individuals. Tight control of blood pressure, diabetes, asthma, seizure, and other conditions is the responsibility of your primary care physician. Be sure to inform your primary care physician of your scheduled operation, so proper preparation can be undertaken prior to your surgery.

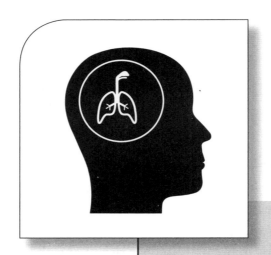

*I have sleep apnea*

# I have sleep apnea

## 35

There are many different kinds of sleep apnea. The most-common form is called Obstructive Sleep Apnea (OSA). This is characterized by interruption of air flow through upper airway passages due to an increased amount of soft tissue or enlarged tonsils. The diagnosis of sleep apnea is made by a sleep study test. Snoring and or a temporary arrest of breathing, morning fatigue and headache, are common features associated with sleep apnea. When the condition is chronic, obstructive sleep apnea may result in high blood pressure and heart failure which may complicate the picture even further. Therefore, a thorough medical evaluation and examination of the airway anatomy are crucial before your scheduled anesthetic.

Patients with sleep apnea are usually very sensitive to intravenous sedatives. Therefore these medications are used very sparingly or in smaller dosages. But inspite of all these precautions many patients with obstructive sleep apnea experience interruption of flow of air when sedated or anesthetized. To address these problems your anesthesiologist has different equipments at his disposal. Obstuction of the air way can be relieved by placement of nasal/oral airways, placement of a breathing tube, or application of the non invasive externally applied airway management device.

At home most patients with sleep apnea, use a breathing assist device called CPAP(Continous Positive Airway Presure). This machine helps flow of air in the airway passeges. You will be asked to bring your CPAP machine with you, especially if you need to be admitted for observation after your procedure and to be available in the recovery room when you wake up from your surgery.

In most cases, you may need to stay in the recovery room longer than usual for close monitoring of your breathing after your anesthetic.

*Redheads and anesthetic requirements*

# Redheads and anesthetic requirements

# 36

Approximately 1% of the human population has red hair. Medical research in the past few years has revealed that people with red hair are potentially more sensitive to pain and may require more anesthesia for their surgical procedure than people with other hair colors. The color of hair and skin is determined by the levels and types of pigments in the cells. This function is normally regulated by the release of a hormone from the brain. Interestingly, these hormones play a major role in the perception of pain. In patients with red hair, due to a genetic dysfunction, there is a higher than normal levels of these brain hormones, resulting in increased sensitivity to pain and possibly an increase in anesthetic requirements.

So what used to be only an anecdotal observation or a myth has proved to have important medical and anesthetic implications.

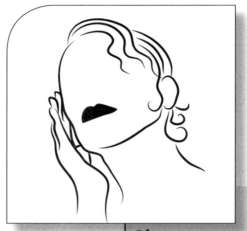

*I have temporomandibular join.*
*(TMJ) problem*

# I have temporomandibular joint (TMJ) problem

## 37

One out of six people suffer from TMJ disorder. It is more common in females and usually is seen in patients between 20-50 years of age. Be sure to inform your anesthesiologist if you suffer from this condition. TMJ disorder may be a problem during your surgical procedure, since during general anesthesia it may be difficult to open your mouth to assist your breathing.

A complete evaluation of your oral anatomy should be performed routinely by your anesthesia provider to assess the extent of your mouth opening and the discomfort associated with the TMJ disorder. This will provide valuable information on how to assist your breathing under anesthesia. In severe cases of TMJ, headache or jaw discomfort might be a post operative compliant.

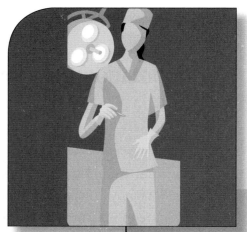

*What if something goes
wrong during my surgery?*

# What if something goes wrong during my surgery?

## 38

The operating room team is composed of a group of highly trained and very skilled individuals, who each specialize in a different area of patient care. This team is made up of registered nurses, surgical technicians, surgeons and anesthesiologists.

Just like a group of musicians brilliantly performing a musical masterpiece, this team is equipped and prepared to respond and treat any unforeseen complications and emergencies that may arise during your surgery. This may be a problem with the normal beating of the heart, a flare up of a pre-existing asthma condition, sudden excessive bleeding or any other problems that may arise during surgery.

In most cases, the anesthesiologist is the director and commander in chief during these hectic situations, as they are trained to respond and treat sudden and acute medical and surgical emergencies. Vigilance and attentiveness to monitoring almost every bodily function are the reasons behind the tremendous improvement in surgical and anesthetic outcomes.

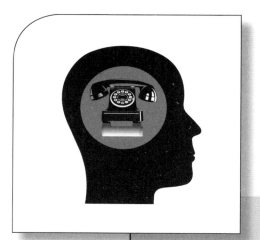

*Who will update my family while I am under anesthesia?*

# Who will update my family while I am under anesthesia?

## 39

Adjacent to every operating theater there is a designated area staffed with a volunteer desk that will accomodate your family members while you are being cared for. In most cases an operating room nurse will update your loved ones periodically of the progress of surgery. These updates will usually inform them of start of the procedure, a surgical progress report, and finally informing your family of conclusion of the procedure along with your general conditions at that time. Once the operation is finished and while you are recovering in the post anesthesia care unit, the surgeon will meet with your family and will provide them with the results of the operation and will answer any questions they may have at that time.

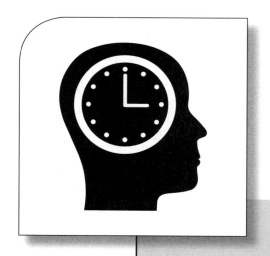

*Duration of surgery*

# Duration of surgery

## 40

The duration of surgery depends on the type of procedure, unexpected problems during the operation, and on your surgeon. There are important anesthetic and surgical implications associated with the duration of surgery. These among other things can include increased risk of infection, possible increased blood loss, and a drop in body temperature. To compensate for these potential problems, usually repeat doses of antibiotics are administered to prevent infections. Electrical warming blankets and intravenous fluid warmers are used to keep the body temperature near normal, and if the blood count drops below acceptable levels, you may need to receive a blood transfusion.

For these reasons, every effort is made to increase the efficiency of the surgical team in an effort to cut down on the length of stay in the operating room.

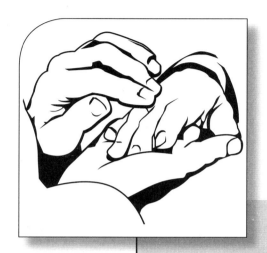

*The recovery room*

# The recovery room

## 41

The recovery room or the post anesthesia care unit is the area designated to take care of you after your surgery. Usually a highly skilled nurse specialized in this field will care for you in the recovery room. Your anesthesiologist is readily available to attend and to make sure the pain is well taken care of and other common post operative problems, such as nausea and vomiting, are controlled. You will be closely monitored to make sure your vital signs are within normal limits. Usually supplemental oxygen is administered to you with either a mask or nasal cannula. Normally family members are not allowed in the recovery room. But some healthcare facilities allow parents to be present as their young child is recovering from surgery and anesthesia. The average length of stay in the recovery room is about one hour.

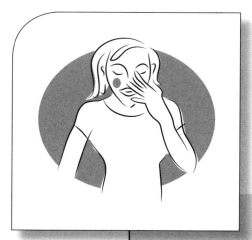

## Nausea and vomiting after anesthesia and surgery

# Nausea and vomiting after anesthesia and surgery

## 42

Nausea, vomiting and pain are the most common side effects one may experience after surgery and anesthesia. Up to 30% of patients may experiece post operative nausea and vomiting. The following factors may increase the risk of post operative nausea and vomiting:

1-Female gender

2-Obesity

3-History of nausea and vomiting after previous procedures

4-Pain

5-Type of the surgical procedure. Some surgeries are associated with a higher incidence of post operative nausea and vomiting. These include testicular surgeries, surgeries on female organs, eye muscle and middle ear surgeries.

6-Not fasting long enough before the surgery

7-Anesthetic medications (such as laughing gas and narcotic medications)
8-History of motion sickness

Be sure to inform your anesthesiologist if you have a history
of nausea and vomiting after surgeries. Fortunately, there
are numerous effective medications available that can prevent or treat nausea and vomiting associated with surgery
and anesthesia.

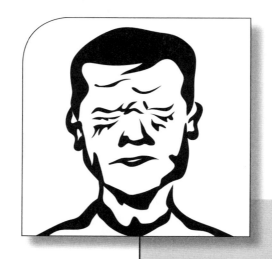

*Pain after surgery*

# Pain after surgery

## 43

Pain is one of the most dreaded consequences of many surgical procedures and is usually due to tissue injury.

Fortunately, nowadays there are numerous ways of preventing and even completely eliminating this feared accompaniment of surgery. Depending on the type of procedure and co-existing medical conditions, spinal or epidural anesthesia may be the best approach to prevent and treat postoperative pain. In addition, different kinds of nerve blocks can also provide adequate pain relief to that area of the body where surgery will be performed. Also, numerous medications can be taken orally or intravenously to kill the pain. Prior to your planned surgery, ask your anesthesiologist about the different pain management options available.

Contrary to common belief, a short course of narcotic pain killers will not result in addiction. Actually, in most cases, narcotics are the cornerstone of an effective pain management regimen.

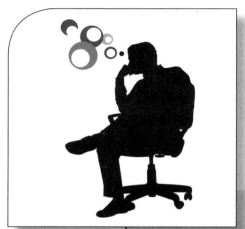

*I am afraid of addiction if narcotics are used for pain control*

# I am afraid of addiction if narcotics are used for pain control

## 44

A short course of treatment with narcotic medications for pain control is considered not addicting and to be generally safe as one of the most effective pain management regimens.

So, don't shy away from these medications as they are also, in most cases, well tolerated.

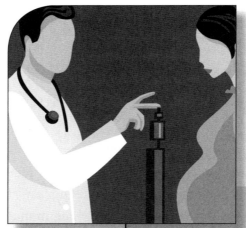

*Pain control during labor and delivery*

# Pain control during labor and delivery

## 45

Epidural anesthesia gives a whole new life to pregnant patients in labor, and the anesthesiologists are your best friend in these trying times.

Like any other medical procedure, when performed properly, epidural anesthesia is usually very safe. In 5 minutes or less after its placement, it will drastically alleviate pain associated with labor.

To perform an epidural anesthetic, you need to be either sitting up or lying on your side. It only takes a few minutes to perform, and the results are dramatic. During this procedure, usually a tiny plastic catheter is placed in your back, which is used to continuously infuse local anesthetics into the epidural space, to control the pain associated with labor and delivery. The bonus is that if you shall need a Caesarian section to deliver your child, the existing epidural catheter is usually adequate for providing anesthesia for this procedure as well.

Epidural anesthesia is safe because the rate of absorption of the medication needed to provide epidural anesthesia is so small that it will not impact the baby.

.

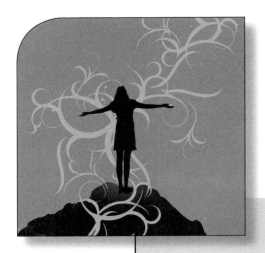

*Dreaming under anesthesia*

# Dreaming under anesthesia

============================================================ **46**

Dreaming under anesthesia is a rather common condition. Dreams experienced under anesthesia are usually similar to those during normal sleep and are usually pleasant, and their content is not related to the surgical procedure. The similarities between the patient's dreams while under anesthesia and during natural sleep suggest that the dreams during anethesia occur during the early recovery period, when you are still lighly sedated but in a definitive sleep state.

Patient characteristics associated with dreaming during anesthesia include; younger age, male, and frequent recall of dreams when sleeping at home. It is also more common when surgery is performed under spinal anesthesia.

You should be reassured that dreaming under anesthesia is not a sign of inadequate depth of the anesthetic.

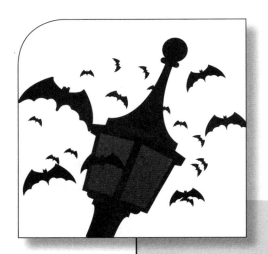

*Nightmares after anesthesia*

# Nightmares after anesthesia

## 47

Unfortunately, some patients report experiencing night-mares after their anesthetic. The incidence is higher in patients with pre-existing psychological disorders. Also, there is a higher incidence of nightmares when certain anesthetics medications are used.

Nightmares are also a very rare but unfortunate complication after surgery even when despite evidence of adequate depths of anesthesia, the patient still had some degree of awareness of intra-operative events. In this case, nightmares could be a reflection of subconscious response to the trauma of being aware under anesthesia. In this rare but unfortunate instance, a psychiatric consultation is warranted and every effort should be made to support the patient emotionally and psychologically.

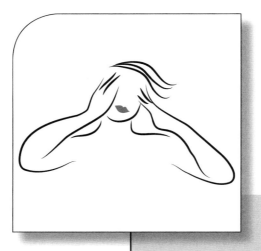

*Headache after anesthesia*

# Headache after anesthesia

## 48

Headache is a relatively common postoperative problem, especially after general anesthesia. Headaches may be a sign of caffeine withdrawal in a patient who is a high caffeine consumer. But in most cases, it is an exacerbation of a pre-existing headache condition such as migraines. However, there are no hazards when anesthesia is administered to patients with this disorder. Sometimes you may experience a headache after spinal or epidural anesthesia. The headache is worse if you stand or sit but is mostly relieved when you lie down. This is called a spinal headache and is due to leakage of spinal fluid into the surrounding tissues at the insertion site of the spinal or epidural needle. Normally, the spinal fluid circulates around the brain and the spinal cord and helps maintain the brain in a floating position when we are standing or sitting up. In the absence of an adequate amount of spinal fluid, due to leakage at the needle insertion site, the brain begins sagging, hence, the spinal headache. Usually bed rest, oral pain killers, and drinking plenty of liquids, especially caffeinated beverages, may solve the problem. But the definitive cure is a procedure called a BLOOD PATCH, which is immediately curative. BLOOD PATCH is basically injecting a small amount of your own blood in the same area where the spinal or epidural anesthesia was performed. The injected blood will form a clot and patch the hole created by the spinal or the epidural needle, preventing further leakage of spinal fluid and thus curing the headache. Another medical procedure which may result in headache is electroconvulsive(ECT) or shock therapy which is used in the treatment of major depression. The procedure is performed under general anesthesia and takes only few seconds to perform. In this situation the headache is probably due to contractions in facial and scalp muscles that occur during the therapy, and resolves spontaneously in few hours.

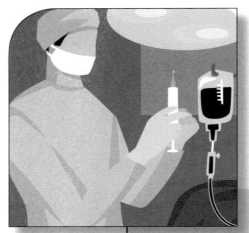

*Blood loss and blood
transfusion*

# Blood loss and blood transfusion

## 49

Different types of surgical procedures will result in varying degrees of blood loss. In some instances there is no bleeding whatsoever. It is important to know your blood type, however in every case the health care facility will recheck to verify this information. If you are scheduled for a procedure, a few weeks in advance you may donate your own blood to be used if blood transfusion becomes necessary during or after surgery. If you do not require transfusion, your donated blood will be added to the pool of blood available in the blood bank to be used for other patients. Other forms of blood product transfusions are also available, such as plasma, platelet or coagulation factor transfusions.

If you are a Jehovah's Witness, it is imperative to inform your health care provider during your first visit so that proper documentation is added to your medical records. Some even advocate for medical alert bracelet for Jehovah's

Witnesses in case of an emergency situation, such as unconsciousness due to a motor vehicle accident so that the patient's wishes regarding blood transfusion are honored.

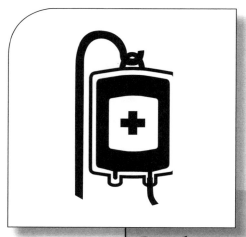

# Complications of
# blood transfusion

# Complications of blood transfusion

## 50

Anesthesiologists are the most likely physicians to administer blood products. Blood transfusion may become necessary if there is a significant blood loss during surgery, jeopardizing normal and vital bodily functions such as adequate blood flow to the brain, heart and kidneys. If major blood loss is anticipated before your procedure, a blood test is performed to determine your blood type, so that an adequate amount of blood is available for your surgery. If you are 2-3 weeks away from your scheduled operation, you may even donate your own blood, to be used if transfusion becomes necessary during or after your surgery.

The risk of life-threatening complications after transfusion is very rare and is less than the risk of death in a motor vehicle accident. Blood products are usually refrigerated, and unless a blood warmer is used during the transfusion process, one of the complications of transfusion could be a drop in body temperature or hypothermia, resulting in shivering in the recovery period after your surgery.

Fever may also be a manifestation of transfusion reaction. This occurs approximately in 1% of those receiving transfusion. In this case, a slower transfusion rate and using medications to treat the fever are all that is needed.

One of the most feared complications of transfusion is the possible transmission of viral diseases such as HIV or hepatitis. In the past few years due to improvement in screening and the testing of donors and blood products, the risk of transmission of HIV has dropped significantly.

The most feared complication of transfusion happens when the wrong blood type is given to you. This may result in kidney shutdown and multiple organ failure. But signs and symptoms of this condition are so dramatic that it results in immediate discontinuation of transfusion and implementation of treatments to support and protect kidneys and other vital organs.

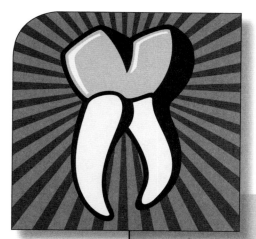

*Dental injury due to anesthesia*

# Dental injury due to anesthesia

## 51

Anesthesiologists are also known as "masters of the airway." Whenever you under go any type of anesthetic or sedation, even in the twilight state, your anesthesia provider may need to assist, and or support your breathing one way or another. Any of these procedures carry a risk, albeit very small, of dental trauma. So a very loose tooth may become dislodged, or a permanent tooth may be chipped. It is worth emphasizing, that in the hands of trained professionals these complications are extremely rare. To safeguard against these complications, bite blocks and or tooth guards are used to protect your teeth. As a means of prevention, your anesthesiologist routinely performs a complete evaluation of your oral anatomy and the condition of your teeth prior to the procedure. Remember, for most procedures it is required for dentures to be removed prior to the administration of anesthesia, especially if the procedure is performed under general anesthesia.

In rare instances when a dental trauma has occurred, a dental consultation is requested (if the healthcare facility has a dentist on staff), or you will be referred to a dentist on an outpatient basis.

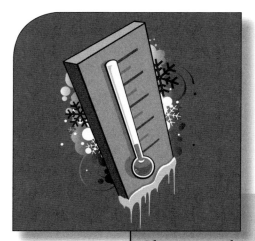

*Shivering after anesthesia*

# Shivering after anesthesia

================================================ **52**

Shivering is a very unpleasant sensation after surgery. Postoperative shivering usually occurs for two reasons: exposure to cold operating room environment and receiving cold intravenous fluids that, in most cases, are kept at room temperature (cooler than your body temperature). So, the longer your surgery takes, the cooler your body becomes and after surgery this presents itself as shivering.

A drop in body temperature has important anesthetic and surgical implications. Hypothermia may be associated with increased risk of bleeding, higher than normal incidence of infection, slow awakening from anesthesia, and it may even delay healing of the surgical wound. Therefore, nowadays every attempt is made to keep your body temperature near normal. This is achieved by using warmed intravenous fluids, warming blankets, or increasing the temperature in the operating room. If postoperative shivering is a problem, a

small dose of some narcotics and usage of electrical warming blankets, in most cases, resolves the problem.

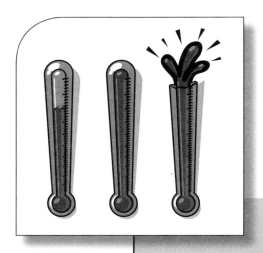

*Fever after anesthesia*

# Fever after anesthesia

## 53

The most common cause of fever after surgery and anesthesia is infection. Blood transfusions and an overactive thyroid can also produce fever after anesthesia and surgery. Fever can be one of the signs of a rare, but very serious complication of general anesthesia. This is called Malignant Hyperthermia (MH). It may manifest itself immediately, or within 24-48 hours after your anesthesia, as stiff muscles, fever and agitation. MH is a medical and anesthetic emergency. Any health care facility that provides general anesthesia is required by law to be equipped with the specific medications necessary for the treatment of MH.

Malignant Hyperthermia is an inherited condition, making these individuals susceptible to this complication when certain anesthetic medications are used to provide anesthesia. Be sure to inform your anesthesiologist if yourself or a family member has been afflicted with MH, as avoidance of certain anesthetic medications will prevent this complication during surgery.

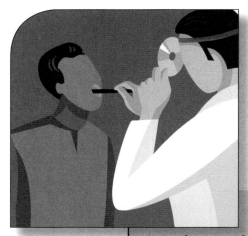

# Sore throat after anesthesia

# Sore throat after anesthesia

====================================================== **54**

This complication of anesthesia is more common when a breathing tube is placed during general anesthesia. The purpose of the breathing tube (Endotracheal tube) is to assist your breathing during surgery and also to prevent stomach secretions from entering your lungs.

A young female patient is more prone to this complication because of more delicate tissue in the air passages. This problem, in most cases, is mild and self limiting, lasting between 24-48 hours and invariably responds favorably to sore throat lozenges.

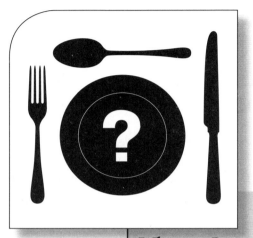

*When can I eat after my surgery?*

# When can I eat after my surgery?

====================================================55

The resumption of oral intake depends on the type of your surgery and type of anesthetic. If you had a minor procedure, such as cataract surgery or breast biopsy under sedation and local anesthesia, you can start oral intake soon after the end of the procedure, usually before you are discharged. But when the procedure is more complicated, especially when it involves the gastrointestinal tract, or if you had general anesthesia for your surgery, at least several hours must elapse before resumption of oral intake is allowed.

Invariably, the start of oral intake is with clear liquids and if tolerated well, can be advanced to small portions of solid foods like crackers. Overeating immediately after your procedure may make you feel sick to your stomach. This especially happens during the ride home as movement alone, particularly in patients prone to motion sickness can cause nausea and vomiting.

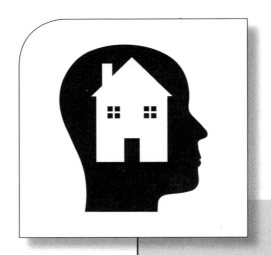

*When can I go home?*

# When can I go home?

This depends on type of the procedure and type of anesthetic. For example, if you had a minor procedure under local anesthesia and sedation, such as cataract surgery, colonoscopy, breast biopsy or MRI procedures, it is OK for you to go home soon after termination of the procedure, assuming your vital signs are stable. Keep in mind that you have to make arrangements for your transportation, as you are not allowed to drive yourself home.

However, if your surgery was more involved, such as back or bowel surgery, you may need to stay for few days in the hospital. This allows time for continued antibiotic therapy and pain management and a more in-depth evaluation of the results of the surgical procedure.

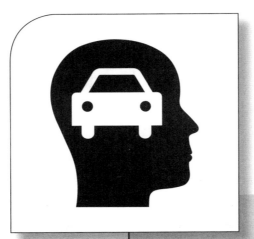

*I don't have anyone to take me home after my surgery*

# I don't have anyone to take me home after my surgery

=**57**

You need to be accompanied by a family member or a friend, as you are not allowed to drive yourself home after you have had anesthesia. If you don't have anyone to help you in that regard, the hospital can make arrangements for transportation by calling a cab, or in some instances, the hospital may even have its own transportation services.

If you live alone and need assistance during your recovery from surgery, the hospital may provide home healthcare services, or you may be discharged to a rehab or extended care facility until you have recovered fully and are able to function independently.

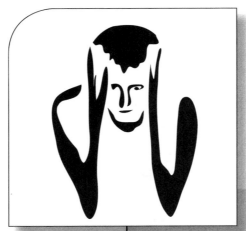

*What if I don't feel well when I go home?*

# What if I don't feel well when I go home?

## 58

Basically you will not be discharged from the health care facility until you meet certain discharge criteria, which are not limited to stable blood pressure, acceptable oxygen levels, reasonable control of your pain level and lack of nausea and vomiting.

Almost invariably the most common complaint at home is pain and or nausea and vomiting. Rarely bleeding is the problem. I strongly advise never to assume that it is OK to have some kind of post-operative problem. You need to call your surgeon's office and alert them to your situation. In some cases, immediate medical attention may be necessary. So, play it safe and consult your health care provider if you don't feel well after your surgery.

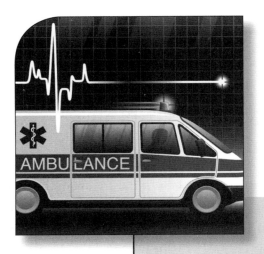

*Emergency surgery*

# Emergency surgery

## 59

In this situation, there is not enough time for fasting and optimizing your bodily functions prior to surgery. However it is reassuring to know that your anesthesiologist and surgical team are always ready to respond to different kinds of emergencies and life or death situations. But one should appreciate the fact that emergency surgeries carry a higher risk of complications, mainly due to the acuteness of the underlying disease process, but also due to a lack of optimization of co-existing medical condition.

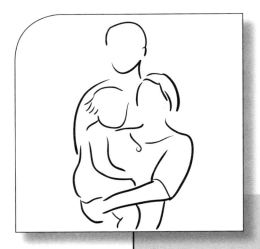

*Anesthesia and my child*

# Anesthesia and my child

## 60

It is astonishing that regardless of age, the thought of anesthesia and surgery provokes the same human reaction. The only difference is that adults fear "not waking up from anesthesia" while children have a fear of pain and separation from their parents. This fact is more pronounced in children between the ages of 1-6 years old.

The best way to alleviate the fear and anxiety related to surgery and anesthesia is to establish a warm physician-patient relationship. Your anesthesiologist can simplify and explain the anesthetic process in an age-related fashion. But, sometimes the level of apprehension is so high that to calm the child and make the process of separation less traumatic, oral medications are used to provide amnesia and sedation. Even with all these steps, as your child is being taken to the operating room, the separation anxiety may still be a problem.

Therefore, some centers allow the presence of parents in the operating room at the beginning of the induction of anesthesia and in the post-anesthesia care unit, where your child is recovering from the procedure.

One of the most frequently asked questions by parents is the duration of fasting prior to the surgical procedure. The minimum fasting period is as follows:

1-Clear liquids (water, pulp-free juices), 2 hours

2-Breast milk, 4 hours

3-Infant formula, 6 hours

4-Solid food, 6 hours

Contrary to adults, the start of an intravenous acess is not usually necessary with children as anesthesia is induced by inhalation of the anesthetic gases.

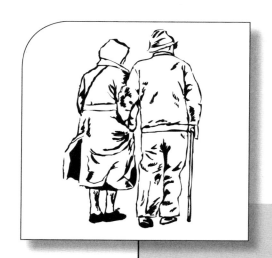

*Aging and anesthesia*

# Aging and anesthesia

## 61

It is a known medical fact that the older we get, especially after 65-70 years of age, the risk of anesthetic and surgical complications increases. The reason is that with aging, there is a general decline in the overall function of all organ systems and therefore more chance to be afflicted with diseases like hypertension, diabetes and lung problems, which can complicate the anesthetic procedure.

Additionally, psychological concerns may be intensified by the fear of loss of function and independence as a result of anesthetic complications. The decline in brain and nervous system function that accompanies aging results in increased sensitivity to anesthetics. Therefore, sedative medications normally used for relieving anxiety should be used sparingly as their effects may be prolonged. Temporary mental dysfunction, presenting as confusion and disorientation, is one of the most common complications in the elderly following anesthesia and surgery.

It is imperative to provide your health care professional with a complete medical history, the list and the dosage of your medications, and whether there have been any complications with previous anesthetics.

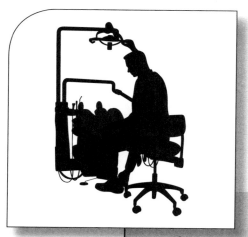

*Anesthesia and dental procedures*

# Anesthesia and dental procedures

## 62

Most dental procedures can be safely and reliably performed under local anesthesia. But in some instances the dentist may need to put you to sleep using either intravenous sedation or nitrous oxide, commonly known as "laughing gas." You need to be certain that your dentist has had proper training and is certified in providing this type of anesthesia. It is even prudent to ask if the office is equipped with resuscitation equipment and if there are policies and procedures in place for transferring patients to a hospital in case of an emergency.

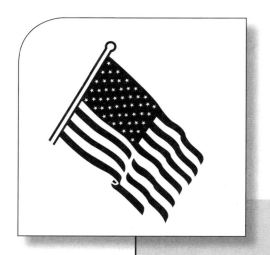

*I don't speak English*

# I don't speak English

## 63

Most health care facilities have interpreters on site (usually employees in different departments) that may be called for communication assistance. Most patients who don't speak English may choose to call a friend or a family member who can be called  to act as interpreter. Of course, making these arrangements in advance makes life easier for everyone.

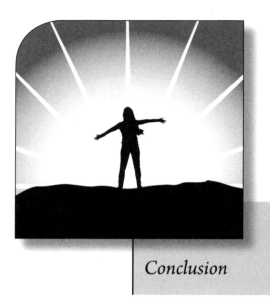

*Conclusion*

# Conclusion

In conclusion, I hope you found the answers to your questions and comfort within the sentences and chapters of this book. Marie Curie once said; "Nothing in life is to be feared. It is only to be understood."

As we make progress in our knowledge and understanding in the field of anesthesiology, one objective remains constant, and that is to provide you with a safe and smooth transit through your anesthetic and surgical experience.

***Anesthesiology is an art, and it is the key to successful surgery.***

# Glossary

**Anaphylaxis:** A severe life threatening allergic reaction

**Antibodies:** Proteins found in blood stream as part of the immune system to neutralize foreign bodies and germs

**Antihistamines:** Medications used in prevention or treatment of allergies

**Anxiolytic:** Medications used in the treatment of anxiety

**Biopsy:** A surgical procedure to obtain a small piece of tissue

**Blood patch:** A procedure used to treat spinal headache

**Caesarian section:** A surgical technique used to deliver the child

**Cardiac:** Related to the heart

**Claustrophobia:** A fear of confined spaces

**Cochlear implants:** An electric device implanted surgically in the ear to help patients with severe hearing deficit

**CPAP:** Continuous Positive Airway Pressure, a device used to help the sleep apnea process

**CT-Scan:** Computerized Tomography: A radiological technique to visualize detailed structures of the body

**DNR:** Do Not Resuscitate

**EKG:** Electrocardiogram, a device used to trace the electrical activity of the heart

**Endotrachael tube:** A tube placed in the trachea used for delivery of oxygen and anesthetic gases to the patient

**Implants:** Any foreign body or device implanted surgically in the body

**MRI:** Magnetic Resonance Imaging, An imaging technique used to visualize detailed structures of the body

**Narcotics:** A class of medications used to control pain

**Nasal cannula:** A delivery system for oxygen via a small plastic tube placed in the nose

**Nerve root:** The initial part of the nerve as it leaves the spinal cord

**Pigment:** The material in the human or animal cell that provides color to that cell

**Postsurgical:** After surgery

**Presurgical:** Before surgery

**Preterm labor:** Start of labor before 37 weeks of pregnancy

**Pulmonary:** Related to the lungs

**Recovery room:** The area where you recover from anesthesia

**Sleep apnea:** A disorder characterized by pauses in breathing during sleep

**Spinal space:** The space in vertebrae through which spinal cord passes

**TemporoMandibularJoint(TMJ):** The joint between the skull and the jaw bones

**Trimester:** One of the three periods of pregnancy each lasting three months

**Twilight anesthesia:** Anesthesia performed under sedation

**Vital signs:** Referring to your blood pressure, heart rate, temperature, rate of breathing

# Index

BEFORE YOU GO UNDER *is an attempt to alleviate the fear and anxiety related to the anesthetic experience.*

*We believe this can only be accomplished by increasing the knowledge and understanding of the general public regarding the seemingly unknown and conspicuous world of anesthesia, So after reading this book please visit our web site at* **beforeyougounder.com** *and provide us with your feedback.*

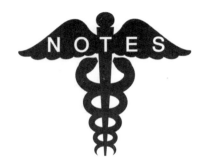

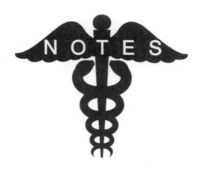

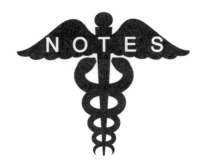